# WATCH YOUR MOUTH!

# WATCH YOUR MOUTH!

Better Health Starts Here

Kevin T. Prince DMD, MPH

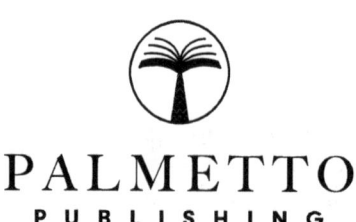

© 2024 Kevin T. Prince, DMD, MPH

All rights reserved.

This book or any portion thereof may not be reproduced or used in any manner whatsoever without the express written permission of the publisher except for the use of brief quotations in a book review.

Paperback ISBN: 979-8-8229-4776-4

*I dedicate this book to my loving wife, Renita, and my son, Kevin Jr. (KJ), for their forever-lasting love and support. You inspire me and motivate me, by your presence in my life, to continue expressing my creative side through your own examples of strength, perseverance, courage, determination, and creativity. My love for you both will far outlast my existence on the planet. It feels so good with you by my side. How pleasant it is to find purpose in our unity.*

# PREFACE

Good health is worth more than diamonds and pearls; there are no manufactured material things in our world that can buy you good health. There are and have been thousands of super-wealthy people in our world who are currently suffering or have in the past suffered with poor health, and all the wealth and access to wealth in the world cannot or could not change their fate. Good health is the money we use to purchase a good life filled with aspirations, hope, faith, and happiness.

## LONGEVITY IS NOT ENOUGH!

As the great architect of the universe would have it, everything must change; nothing stays the same. In his 1977 recording of "Everything Must Change," lyrics by Benard Ighner, George Benson sings, "Everything must change; nothing stays the same. Everyone must change; nothing stays the same. The young become the old, mysteries do unfold…there are not many things in life you can be sure of except rain comes from the clouds, and sun lights up the sky, and hummingbirds do fly. Winter turns to spring; wounded hearts will heal…' Cause that's the way of time; nothing and no one goes unchanged" (Ighner 1977). If our creator grants you any extended time on the planet, you will change over time, and there is not enough Botox or plastic surgery to prevent the change in your physical appearance or your mental sharpness. Yes, we all desire to live a long life. Longevity brings unrevealed value to the things that we cherish most in our world. I would argue that longevity absent quality of life brings little, if any, added value or joy to our human existence. For example, if you live to be ninety-three years old and the last twenty-three years of your life are spent lying in bed unable to move and take care of your basic human needs without a caregiver, I ask is that the quality of life that you were envisioning in your mind?

## QUALITY OF LIFE MATTERS

What really matters, in the end, is the quality of your life on our planet. For each of us, our individual journeys here are limited in the grand scheme of things, and we must do what is in our control to stay physically, mentally, and spiritually as healthy as we can for as long as we can. Father Time is undefeated, and we all will eventually take a knee to our time on the planet, but while we are still here, it is incumbent upon each of us to put in the work required to improve and maintain some portion of good health according to our own human existence. We as humans have little control over how long we will be on this earth, but what we can control is the quality of our existence. That includes the healthy choices that we make, such as the foods we eat and the physical activity we make a part of our daily lifestyle. We as humans must show that we can marry our thirst for longevity with our desire for a good overall quality of life. Only then can we realize the true gift of our human existence. Yes, we are living longer because of the advances in medical technology, medicines, and vaccines, but as our length of stay on the planet may be improving, the overall quality of our existence can only improve through the food choices and life choices that we make. Good health really does begin in the mouth and the choices we make about what we put in our mouths. As a dentist, I am always encouraging other healthcare professionals, such as physicians, physician assistants, nurses, and nurse practitioners, to look into the patient's mouth—preventive dentistry does not require a dental degree or dental chair. It is important for other health-care professionals to make the connection between oral health and general health to provide more holistic care for our patients. My ongoing interest in the collective health of the human population inspired me to earn my master's in public health during my military service. The goal for our human journey on the planet should be what I call "Long Qual" or "LQ." LQ requires us to seek what is pure, raw, and untarnished about our human existence. With LQ, we are relentless and demanding about achieving the things that bring value, nourishment, and purpose to our lives. With LQ, we reject the things that degrade us, dehumanize us, and destroy our souls. LQ means finding quality in our longevity and a sense of longevity in the quality of life that we build through self-actualization.

My hope is that this book will aid in opening our minds to the power that we have to create a healthier earth time for ourselves. Hippocrates once said, "The greatest medicine of all is to teach people not to need it" (Hippocrates 2024). Cheers! To a long life filled with quality and purpose built on a durable foundation of good physical, mental, and spiritual health.

# CHAPTER 1:

# SALT
## (SODIUM)

Adding "taste" to a dish or recipe often means adding salt (sodium) or other spices high in sodium to the food being prepared. Adding sodium to our food without ever tasting the dish beforehand is not unusual. Too much sodium in the human diet can lead to serious health conditions, such as high blood pressure, which could increase your risk for stroke and cardiovascular (heart/circulation) problems.

The ultra-processed foods on our grocery aisles are exceedingly high in sodium. The food manufacturers often add significant amounts of salt and sugar to their products to make them taste good. Oftentimes, when a food manufacturer labels a food product as low sodium, they raise the sugar content in that product to keep a certain level of taste. In a product marketed as "low sugar," often the salt content is increased to keep the taste of the product. Bottom line, be careful and read the nutrition label for those products marketed as low sodium or low sugar. Normally one or the other of these two ingredients is raised to make up for the loss of the other.

In a large number of soul food vegetable dishes, portions of pork or other meats are regularly used to season the vegetables—collard greens, cabbage, and others. These added meats also raise the salt content of these soul food dishes significantly.

For African Americans, Latinos, Native Americans, and other racial and ethnic minority groups in the United States, the health disparities are significant when compared to white Americans. In the United States, there are socioeconomic, environmental, historical, and health-care system issues that contribute to these health disparities. African Americans and other minority groups in general must be mindful of lowering their sodium intake daily. This will help to lower elevated blood pressure and prevent unwanted health problems, including heart and kidney disease, strokes, and other ailments.

Two effective ways to help lower your blood pressure and improve your kidney function while also lowering your sodium intake are to eat more fruits and vegetables high in potassium and drink a minimum of eight full glasses of water per day. Consumption of bananas and green leafy vegetables that are high in potassium, along with raising your daily water intake, will help to regulate your blood pressure. The increased water intake will help to dilute and moderate the sodium levels in your bloodstream. It can also help to lubricate your joints and flush potentially harmful impurities from your body.

Do a comparison next time you go shopping. Compare the regular brand of the product to the low sodium brand and see if you can tell the difference in the amount of sugar and fat content added.

Usually when something is not tasty enough, the first thing we do is reach for the saltshaker, and when something is not sweet enough, we reach for the sugar.

Excessive sodium in your bloodstream can potentially lead to hypertension or high blood pressure, which, if left untreated, leads to other complications, like stroke, kidney disease, and other health problems. Too much sodium in your food can be toxic and will lead to serious health problems if not brought under control. Pay close attention to the amount of salt that you take in daily and take steps to keep your sodium intake below the recommended daily allowance. A diet high in salt can cause retention of fluids, which in turn may raise blood pressure levels. It is best to keep your salt intake to less than 2,300 milligrams a day or one level teaspoon of salt. If you're fifty-one or older, you are African American, or you have high blood pressure, diabetes, or chronic kidney disease, it is important to keep your salt intake to 1,500 milligrams or less. To reduce your sodium intake, try eating more whole and homemade foods and swapping the saltshaker for spicy, no-salt herb blends. Alternatives containing potassium, magnesium, and less sodium may also be helpful. Garlic is a great substitute for seasoning food without adding salt. Also, onions, ginger, curry powder, and oregano can add seasoning to your favorite dish without increasing the salt content. Make no mistake about it, the overconsumption of sodium has proven to be detrimental to the general health of African Americans and other racial and ethnic minority groups.

When shopping for food in the grocery store, look for foods that have a low-sodium content per serving size with low saturated fat and low sugar. If you make a concerted effort to pay attention to the nutrition label, it is possible to find foods that meet these criteria. It is possible to find other seasonings besides salt and salt-based spices to season your food with that will enhance the flavor while decreasing your salt consumption.

Having spent my young childhood in public housing, I know that the food deserts or lack of healthy food options in poor and underserved communities is real. This overexposure in poor and underserved communities to fast foods and heavily processed foods that are high in sugar and salt contributes to the health disparities already documented in poorer communities. You are what you eat, and for humans, our food is the first medicine that we ingest. For many African Americans, soul food and southern cuisine are based on the concept of making foods tastier by adding copious amounts of salt and other high-sodium spices for seasoning to give the food that soulful taste. Well, that overindulgence in table salt and table sugar has wreaked as much havoc on the health of African American and other minority communities than any other destructive force people of color have faced within the United States and globally. We have all craved certain foods at times in our life. I can remember saying as a child, "I just got to have some of Big Mama's sweet lemonade, meatloaf, mac and cheese, and pound cake." What I was really saying in those moments is "Bring on the sugar and salt."

The next time you are in the grocery store, pick up any product and look at the food label on that product. What you will find is that sodium or salt is present in every product you pick up in the grocery store with a few exceptions. The key is to figure out the amount of sodium per serving you are consuming. Look on the soup aisle and pick up almost any brand of soup. What you will find is that most soups have a very high sodium content per serving. The same can be said about most packaged foods that you find on the grocery shelf. Ramen noodles are another fitting example of a food you find on your grocery shelf that contains high sodium content per serving. Let me be clear: the human body needs a certain amount of sodium to properly function, so I am not saying that you should not consume sodium. But what I am saying is that you should watch the amount of sodium that you take in daily because, like sodium's cousin sugar, too much of it can be harmful to your health. Please keep in mind, in this world of excess indulgence in which we live, moderation in the foods that we ingest can positively affect our overall health.

Here are proven ways to get your blood pressure down. First, you must reduce and watch closely your daily sodium intake. Avoid as much as possible saturated fats and cholesterol in your foods. Consider these two things detrimental to your good health. Get to moving. Walk, garden, mow the lawn—just move thirty minutes each day. Maintain a healthy weight for your height. Here is a good rule of thumb for both men and women: when you are standing up straight, if you look down and cannot see the toes of your feet, you are probably overweight for your height. The more body fat that you carry around, the harder your heart has to work to pump blood throughout your body. Put down the saltshaker and find other spices that do not contain sodium to use as seasoning for your food.

# CHAPTER 2:

# SUGAR
## (SUCROSE OR FRUCTOSE)

Oh sugar! That sweet-tasting sugar, that addictive sugar, that substance that attracts us all—it captures us and excites our brains. Here is a bit of history about that good old sugar. Sugar is a by-product of the sugarcane plant, which is grown in areas in the United States, the Caribbean, and other places around the world where the climate is warm. As many European nations began sailing around the world, sugar, rum, cotton, and rice became some of the hottest commodities for traders sailing into foreign ports. These European countries—Britain, Spain, Portugal, France, and others—began colonizing the territories where they were sailing their ships to obtain the natural resources more effectively from those parts of the world. They required labor to grow, harvest, and extract those commodities, for selling, trading, and bartering around the globe. Hence the African slave trade earnestly began out of this high demand for laborers. The slave trade was financed by the wealthiest European countries and investment in these hot commodities to ensure that there was enough free labor to grow, harvest, and extract that sugar from the sugarcane plant and the other natural resources, which was at that time very difficult and labor-intensive work.

A few years back, my wife and I took a trip to Jamaica and stayed at a resort that in its past life had been the site of a sugarcane plantation. There were historical pictures at various locations around the resort that showed well-dressed British aristocrats in social gatherings, celebrating the spoils of the Caribbean Island they had colonized. There were also pictures depicting Jamaicans on sugarcane plantations performing the laborious work required to bring that crop to market to sell in Britain, Europe, and other global destinations. You see, the Jamaicans on those sugarcane plantations were direct descendants of the African slaves brought to Jamaica during the slave trade to supply free labor for the colonial rulers of the island country. This kinship of displaced African sugarcane laborers can be found throughout the Caribbean Islands and North America in places like Louisiana, where the climate was ripe for sugarcane plant growth. The exploitation of free and forced African labor made many colonizers and those who funded and supported them around the globe very wealthy.

You are wondering by now why I felt it necessary to provide you with this history about sugar and the exploitation and exportation that it produced globally, and here is my answer. The crystallized white substance that we know as sugar produced historically in many instances by the forced labor of people of color is now having detrimental impacts on the health of people of color in the United States and around the world because of our overconsumption of it. The overconsumption of this crystallized white substance from the sugarcane plant is making us fatter and sicker every day. On average, Americans consumed about ten teaspoons of sugar every five days two hundred years ago. Today, the average American consumes, without knowing, the same amount of sugar every seven hours. Take time to look at the food label during your next visit to the grocery store. Most processed foods, including foods you would be surprised to know about, from processed meats to soups to cereal, have added sugar. In most if not all energy bars, granola bars, and breakfast cereals, sugar is the number one, number two, or number three ingredient.

We will continue to be disappointed by our health-care system's ineffectiveness and rising cost to treat diet-related, preventable chronic diseases. It is imperative that we collectively speak up and speak out about the devastating human health effects of the processed foods and beverages we consume. If you pick up any food product where sugar is one of the first three ingredients, put it down at once and walk away for the sake of your health.

Sugar by any other name is still sugar. The sugar industry manufactures sugar under a variety of different names. If you are not sure about the ingredients that you are seeing on that food label, pull out your mobile phone and look them up. Pause for the cause of eliminating as much processed food and sugar from your diet as possible. Your body and your health will thank you.

Every other commercial on television nowadays is promoting a magical drug to lower the amount of sugar in your bloodstream and secondarily help you to lose weight. There are drugs on the market now used to reduce your A1C that people who do not have a blood sugar problem are using simply because of the drugs' weight-loss effects. What that demand for the drug is doing is making the supply of the drug for diabetics or people who actually have a blood sugar problem scarce and harder to find. The amount of sugar in your blood is commonly known in medical terminology as your A1C.

What is A1C you ask? It is a blood test that measures your average blood sugar levels over the past months. The A1C test is routinely used to diagnose prediabetes and diabetes, and it is the primary test used by your health-care team to help manage your blood sugar. A normal A1C is below 5.7 percent. An A1C of 5.7 to 6.4 percent is considered prediabetes, and 6.5 percent or higher A1C indicates diabetes. Pharmaceutical companies are raking in the money, and no one is educating the public about how to prevent adult-onset or type 2 diabetes. This overconsumption of sugar is putting increased stress on the human pancreas, that organ in your body that produces the hormone insulin, which manages moving the sugar from your bloodstream to the body's cells, where it is used as energy for cell function. Insulin is the blood sugar regulator, and if insulin is absent or in low supply, your blood sugar level will continue to increase without any counterbalance to keep it in check or at a proper level for your particular body type. That leads to a host of medical conditions that can negatively impact your health and well-being.

Sugar is a carbohydrate that our bodies convert into glucose, which is used by every cell in our body for energy. How does sugar affect our health? Sugar found in fruits is called fructose and is considered a natural sugar. Processed sugar, or sugar produced from sugarcane, is called sucrose. It is extracted during processing of the cane plant and is known as refined sugar. Natural sugars are digested by the human body at a slower rate than processed sugars and help to keep our metabolism stable. Natural sugar does not raise our blood sugar level or glycemic index quite as quickly as refined or processed sugar does. But make no mistake about it: overconsumption of natural or refined sugar will raise your blood sugar levels. Here is the problem: the human body is not designed to manage sugar in abundance, and the pancreas, our insulin-producing organ, will eventually become overburdened and malfunction from sugar overload or overconsumption of sugar.

Refined sugar extracted from the sugarcane plant and processed to make the table sugar we see on the grocery shelves is highly addictive and toxic in excessive amounts. Refined or processed sugar is added to a majority of the processed foods you find in the grocery store, including cereals, tomato sauce, jellies, pickles, ketchup, bread, milk, and the list goes on and on.

Take a walk down the cereal aisle in your local grocery store. A majority of the cereals you see on the shelves are highly processed and contain excessive amounts of added sugar and other preservatives. Usually, the cereals found on the top shelf are the versions with less added sugar, preservatives, and other chemicals that are difficult at best to pronounce. Make no mistake about it: most of the products in the grocery store that you find in a box are highly processed and are detrimental to good health. Refined sugars and processed foods are all destructive to human health and can lead to negative health outcomes. Unless the product says, "No sugar added," you can bet there is some amount of added sugar in that product. Even if the product says, "No sugar added," there may be trace amounts from the processing of that product. Keep that in mind.

Most juices that you find on the grocery shelf have added high fructose corn syrup, which is an alternative form of sugar harvested from corn and made from corn starch. The main ingredient in most pancake syrups on the grocery shelf is high-fructose corn syrup or regular corn syrup. Corn syrup is a less costly alternative to sugar, and it is used regularly in highly processed and bulk-produced food like soft drinks, jellies, fruity drinks, and candies. High fructose corn syrup is a highly processed alternative sweetener and a cousin to sugar, and you will find it in lots of foods on your grocery store shelves. The next time that you pick up that sports drink or sports energy bar in the store, take a minute to look at the nutrition label and see the amount of sugar that is added to make that product. You will be surprised.

Obesity and type 2 diabetes have become commonplace in the United States. There should be no wonder why. If the very first ingredient in a product you are about to buy is high fructose corn syrup or sugar, run, don't just walk, away from that product.

Sugar has been extremely destructive in particular communities, and it continues to be significantly impactful, as far as negative health outcomes, in the African American community. African Americans have culturally for generations overconsumed sugar. We have habitually added lots of sugar to our foods, and it has become commonplace to do so when making "soul" food. I cannot recall how many times I, as a kid, bragged about my Kool-Aid-making skills to my friends when all I was simply doing was adding extreme amounts of sugar to the flavored water. As a child, I remember the sweeter the Kool-Aid or lemonade, the better.

The average individual in our country consumes well over the recommended daily amount of sugar. Excess sugar consumption is associated with significant health problems, and this is based on scientific studies and documented in health literature. We as humans like the way we feel when we consume our favorite dessert. Research on brain function has shown that when we eat sugar, certain areas within our brain light up and provide us with a sense of pleasure. Overconsumption of sugar can lead to damaging effects on the human body over time.

As a dentist, over my career, I have seen parents who have unknowingly destroyed their children's first teeth, or baby teeth, by allowing them to consume too much sugar. Some parents nurse their infants or put their infants to bed at night with a bottle filled with milk or another liquid that may have added sugar. Yes, the sugar lights up the pleasure centers in their infant brains, keeping the infant quiet, but it also destroys the infants' teeth. Repeated behavior of supplying sugar-filled drinks over time makes the sugar become more addictive to the infant and causes the infant to be harder to wean off the bottle and quiet down when agitated. Additionally, exposing an infant to excessive sugar during a time when their internal organs are still developing can potentially lead to organ malfunction as they continue to grow, particularly the pancreas, as it produces the all-important hormone insulin, which regulates blood sugar in humans.

Excessive sugar consumption can also cause irreversible damage to our teeth and gums. The millions of bacteria found in the human mouth feed on the sugar that we consume daily. After they consume the sugar from the food that we ingest and the excess sugar found in our bloodstream, the bacteria in our mouth produce an acid by-product. This acid by-product destroys the outer layer solid surface or enamel of our teeth and the bone and gum tissue around our teeth. All of this leads to tooth decay, gum disease, and early tooth loss.

With no teeth to adequately break down the foods we eat and start the proper digestive process in our mouths, we put more strain and work on our stomach and intestines to break down the foods that we swallow to properly absorb the nutrients. With no teeth, we are forced to eat more processed foods that are low in nutritional value and typically high in sugar, salt, and preservatives. This poor diet can lead to even more health issues and problems. Our mouth is the portal of entry to the human body, and human digestion begins in our mouth. The overconsumption of sugar in the human body only acts to accelerate the process of poor health outcomes.

As a practicing dentist and the author of this book, please allow me a moment to opine here. In 1840, some visionary dentists and physicians successfully petitioned the Maryland General Assembly to establish the first organized school of dentistry here in the United States, the Baltimore College of Dentistry. Since that time, the profession of dentistry has worked alongside but outside of the general medical establishment in our country. This has left the impression to the general population over time that the mouth is somehow separate from the rest of the body and that what occurs in the mouth will not have any impact on or relationship to what is occurring in the rest of the human body. I do apologize if you were left with that impression but allow me to correct that bit of disinformation now. Your mouth is an organ system and the main portal of entry to the rest of the human body, and disease or abnormalities identified in your mouth can be a sentinel for disease or abnormalities in the rest of your body. A lot of research being conducted today is exploring the deep connection between oral health and systemic or whole-body health. The more we can unlock and better understand those oral-systemic human body connections, the better future health care we can provide to the population at large. A recent research study on colorectal cancer tumors found significant amounts of oral bacteria in those colorectal tumors. How can that be if the mouth is not connected to the rest of the human body? A report from this colorectal cancer research states,

A bacteria implicated in gum disease, *Fusobacterium nucleatum*, has also been found in some colorectal cancer tumors. F. nucleatum is rarely seen in the guts of healthy people. Colorectal tumors harboring these bacteria are associated with more cancer recurrence and worst patient outcomes than tumors without them, However, it's unclear how much of a role, if any, the bacteria play in causing the tumors to grow. (McMains 2024)

Diabetes is a major health problem in the United States and is particularly pervasive in minority and poorer communities in a variety of racial and ethnic groups. Too much sugar in the human diet raises our blood sugar or blood glucose too high, which leads to diabetes in humans. If your body cannot produce insulin, the sugar you eat builds up in your bloodstream and never makes it into your body's cells where it is used by the body for energy. If your body does not produce insulin, you are considered a type 1 diabetic. If your body produces insulin but not enough to properly regulate your blood sugar, you are a type 2 diabetic. You have what is known as adult-onset diabetes. This is the most common form of diabetes.

Regular exercise, reducing your sugar intake, and eating a well-balanced and healthy diet with an abundance of vegetables and fruits are a few ways that you can lower your risk for complications of diabetes. Some of the complications we see from excess blood sugar or diabetes include heart disease, kidney disease, nerve damage, blindness, stroke, and other health-related problems. Obesity is a major problem in the United States, and problems that affect other racial, ethnic, and minority groups often hit the African American community with triple the effect. Fast foods, soda machines, microwave-ready foods, oversized food portions, and processed meats and meals in a box have all taken over our society and become the norm in American culture. This phenomenon has led to big profits for people promoting these products and manufacturers of these products. A lot of the food that we consume in the American diet is often low in nutritional value and high in the ingredients that make us fatter and sicker over time. With the increase in obesity in this country, we have also seen a rise in adult-onset diabetes. Increasingly younger people are overweight and are becoming diabetic. Younger Americans are consuming more fast foods and ready-made foods. These foods are often filled with excessive amounts of sugar, as well as sodium, saturated fats, preservatives, artificial colors, artificial flavors, and other ingredients that can be harmful to the human body over time. As Americans our waistlines continue getting larger to the detriment of our health. Sugar plays a prominent role in all the madness and poor health outcomes that we are seeing in our culture today. Most physicians recommend that their diabetic patients reduce their sugar intake and exercise more often to help control their blood sugar levels, along with insulin injections as needed.

The next time you pick up one of those sugary drinks, remember you can cut the amount of sugar you are consuming by mixing part of your drink with an equal amount of water. For example, your sugary drink contains twelve grams of sugar in an eight-ounce serving; put four ounces of your favorite drink in a glass and add four ounces of water. This will cut the sugar content of your drink in half, and you will still get that sugar taste that you require and have grown accustomed to while reducing the amount of sugar that you are actually consuming.

As I am completing my work on *Watch Your Mouth*, just last week (April 24, 2024), the United States Department of Agriculture (USDA) announced finalized nutrition guidelines to reduce sugar and salt in school meals.

For the first time, added sugars will be limited in school meals nationwide, with small changes happening by Fall 2025 and full implementation by Fall 2027…Schools will need to slightly reduce sodium content in their meals by Fall 2027…This change still moves our children in the right direction and gives school and industry the lead time they need to prepare. (Agriculture 2024)

This is great news for the future health of our K–12 schoolchildren and if properly implemented will have tangible real-world impact in a shift toward better health for children all over the United States. It amounts to a small but significant step in the right direction.

*Remember, you are what you eat,*
*and your food is the first medicine.*

# CHAPTER 3:

# WATER

If you were stranded in the desert without food or water, which one would you request if you could only have one? I would request water because you can survive much longer on water and no food than on food with no water.

Water, or $H_2O$, is two parts hydrogen and one part oxygen. Because humans have always had an exploratory nature, we are constantly probing space and the galaxy around us, looking for other planets that have any form of life. The main thing we search for on those distant planets is any sign of water. You cannot have water without oxygen, which is a key part, and if you have no oxygen, then human life cannot exist. That is why when astronauts or unmanned rovers visit planets in our solar system, they are looking for signs of life, testing to see if there is oxygen, and searching for traces of water on the planet. Life on planet earth would be unsustainable without water and one of its key components, oxygen.

About seventy-five percent of the human body is made up of water, but if you ask the average American how much water he or she consumes a day, it would be well below the eight glasses of water that most health sources recommend. Water is to the human body what oil is to the engine of a car or plane or any type of mechanical device; it keeps everything lubricated and running as smoothly as possible. The majority of planet earth is water. Do you think that this is a coincidence? Why would the grand architect who set our human existence in motion fill the only planet that humans can inhabit with so much water?

It is difficult to encourage people to drink more water for the betterment of their health if they do not have routine access to clean, potable water for drinking, cooking, bathing, and other everyday tasks. There are environmental, political, socioeconomic, and geographic factors that prevent communities of people from having access to clean drinking water and potable water for everyday use. One of the factors that affects an individual's access to clean and safe water is whether they live in a more urban setting or environment with many people who fall low on the socioeconomic scale. Unless you are living in a cave, you must be aware of the ongoing fight for clean, potable water in mostly urban majority African American communities like Flint, Michigan, and Jackson, Mississippi. A higher percentage of low-income Black and Brown people in our country tend to live in areas where a lack of access to healthier food options (food deserts) exists. Also, due to the decaying infrastructure typically noted in these communities of color, water treatment facilities, if they exist at all, typically have suffered years of neglect. There is also an unwillingness to modernize them based on financial decisions made by local and state politicians who do not live in those communities and often show little concern for the residents who do. What I am speaking about is well documented in our country's history and is known as environmental neglect based on community demographics. Too often these communities of color are found near industrial complexes that put out dangerous and harmful by-products from their manufacturing processes that flow into the air and seep into the soil and eventually the water supply. These pollutants can have a negative impact on the health and well-being of these underserved communities. Therefore, just encouraging people to drink more water to improve their health is shortsighted because drinking more water may be harmful to your health in communities of color if the water you are being asked to consume is brown in color and smells of sulfur or rotten eggs. Yes! Consuming more water is a great message for the populations on our planet that have access to clean, safe, potable water. But what about the other millions of human inhabitants on our planet who may be water deprived? As an advocate for the power of water consumption by humans, I encourage more water intake for human wellness while keeping in mind the lack of access to clean drinking water for millions around the globe.

Water cleanses the human body, water calms our senses, water is cooling, water takes the shape of whatever space it inhabits, and it is present in every cell, muscle, bone, tendon, and organ in the human body. Insufficient water causes toxins like salt and excess sugar to build up in the bloodstream, which can lead to organ damage and organ failure over time. Water is powerful and has the power to reshape our environment through its directional flow and force.

One of the best ways to control your weight is to increase your water intake and decrease the intake of processed foods and sugar-loaded drinks. Water is the best laxative, and if you consume enough, it will keep you regular and help to keep your kidneys functioning properly by flushing out impurities. Your digestive system, liver, lungs, and other organs function more efficiently when properly hydrated with water. One of the best first steps to better health is to consume a large amount of water throughout the day. Water is truly the most important lubricant for human existence.

My challenge to you is to drink more water throughout your day. It will keep your skin looking and feeling healthy and help properly regulate your blood sugar, flush out your kidneys, cleanse your bladder, and promote optimal performance of all your other internal organs. I do recognize for some people just saying to drink more water every day sounds easy, but oftentimes it is a little bit more difficult to do. That is why there are so many flavored waters on the market now to try to encourage people to drink more water. If flavor in your water will make you drink more of it, I say more power to you. Just make sure that flavored water does not have any added sweeteners or sugar.

I am a proponent of drinking alkaline water or what is known as high-pH water. The higher the pH of the water, the better. I normally look for water that is 9.5 pH or higher. Alkaline water with added minerals helps to regulate your digestive flow and is an aid in removing toxins from your body by promoting regular bowel movements and flushing out the kidneys for good urinary flow and excretion of waste. Put down the sweet tea or sweet lemonade and pick up a bottle of water. Your kidneys will thank you for the good flush, and your pancreas will thank you for not making it work overtime to flush out all the sugar in your bloodstream.

*Remember, you are what you eat,
and your food is the first medicine.*

# CHAPTER 4:

# MEAT AND DAIRY

I have often wondered, if you must kill something before you can eat it, should you be eating it at all? This is a question I would ask that you think about as you read this chapter of the book.

The question of whether we were created to be herbivores (plant eaters), or carnivores (meat eaters) is an age-old one. If you follow and believe the biblical teachings, then our creator formed Adam and from Adam created Eve and had them dwell in a garden not on a farm. Why would our creator pick a garden full of plants and trees bearing fruit if the plan were to have man eat other mammals and creatures? If you believe in the humble creation of man by the hands of God, then man's original placement in the garden should lead you to ask the following questions: Did our creator intend for us to eat the plants, fruits, and vegetables produced in the garden? Or did the creator intend for man to consume the other animals on the planet? Or were we created to consume both?

If you choose to be a carnivore or meat eater, I recommend, for your best health outcomes, that you eat the leaner portions of your favorite meat of choice. If you, for instance, are frying chicken, removing all the skin, and cutting away as much fat as possible before frying would give you a leaner portion of animal protein, and if you season and flour it properly, you will not miss the skin of that chicken at all. All your meat products should be washed thoroughly and have as much animal fat and skin removed as possible prior to cooking to avoid the unhealthy fat and the potential microorganisms, which can make you sick and are often found in the skin and fatty layers of your favorite meats. Bottom line, if you are a meat eater, eat the leanest portions of meat that you can buy and cut away the extra fat whenever possible.

If you have issues with high cholesterol, you can reduce the amount of cholesterol in your bloodstream simply by reducing your intake of meat, such as beef, chicken, turkey, pork, and shelled seafood, including crab and shrimp. If you are looking to move to a more plant-based or plant-centric lifestyle, you should gradually remove meat from your current food consumption. Notice I am intentionally not using the word "diet" when it comes to plant-based eating in this chapter, and that is because diets are more faddish and temporary in nature. Transitioning to a plant-based or plant-centric lifestyle requires real commitment and an unwavering determination to change the trajectory of your overall health. Rapid shifts away from a meat-based diet will only serve to frustrate you and lead you to failure in your attempt to transition to a more plant-based lifestyle. What I am saying is that your transition should be gradual and not sudden.

An abundance of the meat consumed in the United States and imported from other countries is often filled with antibiotics, steroids, and other chemicals that are present in animal feed. To keep the animals disease free and help them grow faster so that they can get to the market quicker for human consumption, many farmers and ranchers will use antibiotics and steroids in their animal feed. The Food and Drug Administration, or FDA, is now requiring many meat producers to show on the packaging of their product whether they used antibiotics while growing their animals before the conversion from animal walking around on the farm or ranch to meat products.

A significant amount of the dairy and dairy products in the United States and globally come from cow's milk. All that cheese on your pizza, the butter on your pancakes, and the yogurt in your granola is the product of the body fluid from that renowned farm animal the cow. Yes, the sacred cow produces the beef in the hamburgers that you eat and the milk in your milkshake. If you are lucky, hopefully the soil growing the grass that those cows are eating is not contaminated with pesticides and other chemicals that can potentially find their way into that milk that you are drinking or those beef ribs that you are smoking on the grill. Here is the bottom line: as consumers, we are all heavily dependent on the government and various governmental agencies to ensure that the food we are consuming is in fact safe for human consumption and will not make us sick or, even worse, lead to our demise. Many of the government agencies tasked with food safety are so challenged with staffing shortages and mired in federal regulations that on a good day, they may be unable to adequately provide the oversight, checks, and balances needed to ensure the safety of our food supply. It is scary to think about the fact that one failed attempt at proper oversight of our food manufacturers/producers could have a disastrous effect on the health of the population. If you are a meat and dairy consumer, my advice is to carefully select the quality and amount of meat and dairy you consume, take note of how consumption of meat and dairy makes you feel, and increase your awareness about meat and dairy product recalls.

Diligence and vigilance are extremely important when it comes to the food that you consume. Everything that you eat and drink influences your body. The question is whether the effects of the food and drink that you are consuming are a net positive or a net negative? This is a question you should be continuously asking yourself and reflecting on if you are serious about your journey to a healthier you.

Frequently in the news, we hear about meat recalls because of *E. coli* contamination. *Escherichia coli* (*E. coli*) is a bacterium that normally lives in our intestines. Most types of *E. coli* are of no harm and even work to keep your gut healthy. However, some strains of E. coli can cause intestinal pain and discomfort along with diarrhea if you consume contaminated food or drink polluted water. Processing meat and bringing it to market requires a lot of handling of the product. Each stop in that meat-processing chain of events can lead to contamination of the product and produce sickness in those who consume it. If you are considering moving from a meat-based diet to a more plant-based lifestyle, I would recommend that you look for opportunities to educate yourself about living a plant-based or plant-centric lifestyle. Start your search by looking for vegetarian organizations within your community, and seek out plant-based cooking classes, vegetarian and vegan festivals, and other activities that will introduce you to the plant-based lifestyle.

*Remember, you are what you eat,*
*and your food is the first medicine.*

# CHAPTER 5:

# PLANT-BASED LIFESTYLE

Transitioning to plant-based or plant-centric eating requires a lifestyle change and should never be confused with a fad diet. Becoming a vegetarian or vegan requires a lifelong commitment, and it should not be considered as some meat-free diet you would like to try out every now and then.

Vegetarians avoid meat, fish, and poultry. Those who include dairy products and eggs in their lifestyle are called lacto-ovo vegetarians. A vegan lifestyle is much stricter than the vegetarian lifestyle. Vegans eat no meat, fish, poultry, eggs, or dairy products or anything else that comes from an animal or that is produced by an animal. While there is a considerable advantage to a lacto-ovo vegetarian lifestyle, the vegan lifestyle is the healthiest of all plant-based lifestyles and works along with regular exercise to promote a healthier you. Living a plant-based lifestyle requires resilience and a level of commitment, and I do realize that such a lifestyle is not for everyone. My simple advice is to live your best life now, whether that includes meat, or it doesn't. What I am confident of is that you and I will not pass this way again, at least, not in our current form.

A vegetarian or vegan lifestyle change alone will not help you to lose or control your weight or improve your health by itself. You must—I repeat, you must—incorporate regular physical activity into your plant-based or plant-centric lifestyle change. The wrong plant-based foods can be just as unhealthy for you as a meat eater's diet. Plant-based eating filled with bread, potatoes, rice, and other high-carbohydrate foods can make you just as overweight and unhealthy as someone who is not living a plant-based lifestyle. You must be careful not to get caught up in fad diets and the fast-food cravings that can be found even within the plant-based eating environment. It is imperative that you incorporate what I call clean organic, if possible, plant-based foods into your lifestyle, like spinach, asparagus, mushrooms, and things that have a high nutritional value. In the past couple of years, there have been unique concepts for plant-based fast-food living that have popped up in certain parts of the country. Be very careful. Although these foods may be plant-based, they can be just as unhealthy for you as foods that are not plant-based because of the way they are prepared and because although plant-based, they lack high nutritional value.

Living a true plant-based lifestyle will require a change in the way you view the foods that you eat, a change in how you prepare the foods that you eat, a change in the restaurants that you like to eat in, a change in the way you grocery shop, and a change in the foods that you purchase to eat.

The human body in total is a living, breathing organism and requires food and nutrients that are as close to their original state as possible to fuel the human body and support optimal health. Transitioning to a true plant-based lifestyle will require you to alter your way of thinking about food and its nutritional value. You will have to be more conscious and vigilant about what you put into your mouth and what your body consumes. Things that have no nutritional value only serve to make us more obese and sicker and increase our vulnerability to diseases and the breakdown of the human body.

People living a plant-based lifestyle normally have a much lower cholesterol level than meat eaters. The reasons are that it is not hard to find plant-based meals that are typically low in saturated fat and usually have little or no cholesterol. Cholesterol is typically found in animal products, such as meat, dairy, fish, and eggs. A plant-based lifestyle is typically a low-cholesterol lifestyle. My primary-care physician is normally surprised when they get my blood work back from the lab and notice my low cholesterol level. They usually ask what I am doing to keep my cholesterol level so low. What I always tell them is that I am living a plant-based lifestyle and have noticed that my cholesterol level remains low since I started my plant-based journey over fifteen years ago.

$B_{12}$ is one of the vitamins typically found in a meat eater's diet, so if you are transitioning to a more plant-based lifestyle, it is important that you supplement your food consumption with vitamin $B_{12}$-fortified foods or a $B_{12}$ supplement.

A diet based on vegetables, legumes, fruits, and whole grains that are low in fat and sugar can help lower blood sugar levels. Since individuals with diabetes are at are at a higher risk for heart disease, avoiding fats and cholesterol is important, and a plant-based lifestyle is the best way to avoid unnecessary fat and cholesterol.

A moderate amount of physical activity, as directed by your physician or health-care provider, in conjunction with your newfound plant-based lifestyle will help to make you the healthiest person that you can be.

> *Remember, you are what you eat,*
> *and your food is the first medicine.*

# CHAPTER 6:

# NUTRITION / FOOD LABELS

Good nutrition is a key part of good health. Here are quick notes about food labels. First, I encourage you to take time to read the labels on the food that you pick up to eat. You will be surprised at the ingredients that are in the foods that you and I eat every day. Many of these ingredients you will not be able to pronounce or spell, and more important, you have no idea of the effects these ingredients are having on your body.

I know it may take a few extra seconds of your time, but the only true way to know what is in the foods you are eating is to take time while shopping to read the nutrition label and the list of ingredients. The list of ingredients will tell you generally what is in the food products you are buying. You should know what foods you are putting into your body because that food will affect your overall health. As a general rule of thumb, the more ingredients a food label has on it, the more processed and unhealthier the food is that you are about to consume.

Look for foods that have very few ingredients on the food label. If it is a can of tomatoes, it should have tomatoes as the first ingredient on the label and very few other ingredients. Some of the food labels that you will see in the store have what I call a "chemistry lab" of ingredients on the label. You and I have no idea how this chemistry lab of ingredients will impact our health once we consume that food product.

The next time you are in the grocery store, pick up a bottle of syrup and read the label. You will be surprised how much of every other ingredient besides actual syrup is in that bottle. Normally at the top of the list of ingredients in that bottle of syrup you will find high fructose corn syrup. How does high fructose corn syrup affect your health? Look it up and get a better understanding of what you are consuming. Can you pronounce many of the ingredients? I challenge you to go a step further and look up the ingredients to see what effect they may or may not have on your health. I do like syrup on my pancakes, but I normally buy 100 percent maple syrup. If you read the food label on a jar of maple syrup, you will normally see that the ingredient list is only maple syrup from the maple tree. Oh, even though it's 100 percent maple syrup, please remember it is also sugar, and you should use it sparingly.

I have always believed when it comes to good health, the fewer ingredients that you have in the foods that you consume the better. The more natural a product is the better it will be for your overall health. Therefore, choose healthy food products with fewer added ingredients. Your body will thank you. Take the time to read the label and know what you are putting into your body. Reading and understanding food nutrition labels alone will go a long way to improving your overall health and making you the healthiest person that you can be.

To help you navigate the grocery aisle the next time you are in the grocery store, consider the following it may help you to become a wiser shopper and select healthier food products. It is important to look at serving size when you are reading a food label. The food label on a bag of potato chips may say there are twenty-five milligrams of sodium in the chips that you are considering purchasing. That is the amount of sodium in one serving of chips. However, there may be as many as five servings in that bag of potato chips, so if you eat two servings of the chips, you are consuming fifty milligrams of sodium or twenty-five milligrams for each of the two servings of chips that you consume. Per Food and Drug Administration regulations, if you see the word *light* on a food label for a particular product, that product must have one-third fewer calories than the regular version of the same product. If you see the words *low fat* on a food label for a particular product, that product must have no more than three grams of fat per serving. If you see the words *low in saturated fat* on the food label of a particular product, that product must have no more than one gram of saturated fat per serving and not more than 15 percent of calories from saturated fat. If you see the words *low in sodium* on the food label of a particular product, that product must have no more than 140 milligrams of salt per serving.

Diets just do not work. You must be able to rethink your approach to supporting a healthy weight. It will require a change in basic assumptions and the way you think about your relationship with the foods you consume. The key to achieving and supporting a healthy weight is lifelong good eating and regular routine physical activity. You should not be chasing fad diets. It must be a lifestyle change and requires you to reimagine how you approach healthy living.

*Remember, you are what you eat,*
*and your food is the first medicine.*

# CHAPTER 7:

# EMPTY CALORIES

Empty calories come from foods with no nutritional value that only serve to fill up your stomach without doing anything positive for your overall health. French fries are just one of the fitting examples; the fries will fill up your stomach but have no nutritional value. But the carbohydrates in those potato fries and the oil that the fries are cooked in will expand your waistline. I try to avoid empty-calorie foods as much as possible and usually look for foods that have nutritional value in the way of vitamins, minerals, nutrients, and essential proteins that the body can use to improve function and support good health.

Most empty-calorie foods are high in calories per serving and calories from fat, saturated fat, trans fat, sodium or salt, sugar, simple carbohydrates, and cholesterol. These empty-calorie foods typically have little if any nutritional value.

To cut down on the empty calories, look for foods and snacks that are not hightly processed and have fewer added ingredients, especially if those added ingredients have no nutritional value. Begin to incorporate fresher whole foods into your lifestyle. These are foods that have undergone little if any processing. Processing can strip the foods of their nutritional value. Carrots, kale, raw almonds, raw peanuts, and your fresh fruits and veggies will meet the requirement of unprocessed foods. Keep in mind that overcooking these foods can deplete their nutritional value.

In the world of food and nutrition, brown is better than white. This is quite a statement to make considering we are a society held captive by the burden of color and we live in a world that assigns certain values to color. White breads, pastas, rice, and flour are all made from whole grains that are stripped of their nutritional content during food processing, leaving you with a low-value version of the original product. Brown breads, pasta, rice, and flour are all minimally processed grains and therefore keep their nutritional value with fiber, minerals, and vitamins. The fiber found in these minimally processed grains keeps your stomach fuller longer because of their slow digestion and helps to prevent overeating. Because these minimally processed grains have more complex carbohydrates, they break down more slowly during digestion and tend not to raise your blood sugar quite as fast as the more highly processed simple carbohydrates will do.

For a healthier you, "Be down with brown." If you are hooked on white bread, next time you eat a sandwich, use one slice of white bread and one slice of brown bread, and make the transition to brown gradually. If you like white pasta, mix the white pasta with brown whole-grain pasta, and make the transition to brown gradually. The same goes for rice, flour, and other white grain products.

*Remember, you are what you eat,*
*and your food is the first medicine.*

# CHAPTER 8:

# PHYSICAL HEALTH

Tailor your physical activity to your current state of health and your age. You should consult with your primary-care physician before starting any exercise program. Thirty minutes a day for five to seven days per week is the recommended guidance for regular exercise. I say do not box yourself in with guidelines. Do what fits your lifestyle and your schedule the best. The most important thing is to get up and get active.

Find things that you enjoy doing and that will get you up and moving, and simply do those things more often throughout the week. For you, that may be bike riding, gardening, bowling, tennis, walking, camping, golf, or any other activity that you enjoy doing regularly.

You do not have to be an Olympic athlete to incorporate physical activity into your daily lifestyle. Even a brisk walk in the evening after dinner would be a good start to getting you active. Moderate-intensity activities should be your goal. These include dancing, riding a bike, swimming, gardening—whatever keeps your interest. Just remember whatever you do, it should raise your heart rate and breathing rate and make you sweat a bit for maximum benefit.

During my military service, a height-weight standard was set for both males and females. The goal for service members was to meet the standard to support a healthy weight. You should consult with your primary-care physician or a nutritionist about the proper healthy weight for a person your height and then set a goal of trying to reach and maintain that height-weight balance.

Find a friend who has a similar goal of obtaining and keeping a healthier lifestyle, and motivate each other to help reach your goals. Pray for strength and determination on those difficult days when you are not motivated to exercise and do the things needed to achieve and support good health. It is during those challenging times that you must look deep within yourself for that motivating factor that will get you up and going.

Be realistic and celebrate the small achievements along your journey to better health. Also understand that there may be hills and valleys along your journey to a healthier you. Good health is not about being thin, losing weight, or having your clothes fit better. Good health is about keeping your body in a state of physical, mental, and spiritual well-being all while reaching and keeping a comfortable body weight supportive of your height and your physical stature.

The goal is to reach a level of total well-being; this is different from physical well-being because it also considers your level of mental and spiritual health. Total well-being means having your physical health, mental health, and spiritual health all in sync so that the way you view yourself and the world around you will help to advance your mindset and elevate your state of consciousness as a human being.

Total well-being will help you to see the world with a high degree of optimism and will cause you to surround yourself with like-minded people who are optimistic, purposeful, and health conscious. Healthy people with total well-being want to live in a world that values good health and disease prevention, preserves the environment, and promotes healthy people and communities globally.

You should start your exercise program slowly, especially if you have not been active for a long time. Over time, build up your level of activity and gradually increase how hard you work your body. Remember to warm up your muscles before you begin any exercise routine. A good exercise routine should not hurt or make you feel exhausted. You might feel a little bit of soreness, a little discomfort, or a bit fatigued, but you should not feel pain. The truth is being active will make you feel better as you become more comfortable with your exercise routine and increased physical activity.

*Remember, you are what you eat,
and your food is the first medicine.*

# CHAPTER 9:

# INSPIRATION AND MOTIVATION

Our time on the planet is like a roll of thread unwinding. It is my belief that when we are born, the creator gives each of us a set amount of time to inhabit the planet. How we carry and conduct ourselves through that time will speak to the kind of person that we are and whether "our planet time" has any real purpose. What I am trying to say is do not waste your time waiting for someone or something to motivate you to be a better version of yourself. Others can encourage you, but the true motivation must come from within, so dig deep and find the motivation to start being a better and healthier you right now.

Truth be told, I am working every day to make my limited time here on this planet as healthy and productive as I can. Honestly, there are days I feel like I am winning, and there are days I feel like progress is hard to find. I lean on my spiritual health and faith during those darker times to propel me forward, understanding that the journey is never straight and oftentimes is filled with hills and valleys.

Find your motivation from within yourself, step out on faith, and pray often for guidance and favor from our most omnipotent creator, whose grandness is all-encompassing. Remember your journey to a better and healthier you is not a sprint; it is a marathon, so take that all-important first step forward and watch our creator work. Keep moving toward the goals that you have set. Always remember to pause and celebrate even the smallest victories and milestones along your journey to a healthier you.

> ***Remember, you are what you eat,***
> ***and your food is the first medicine.***

# CHAPTER 10:

# GOOD HEALTH TIPS

According to the Urban Institute, "The number of Americans ages sixty-five and older will more than double over the next 40 years, reaching eighty million in 2040. The number of adults ages eighty-five and older, the group most often needing help with basic personal care, will nearly quadruple between 2000 and 2040" (Institute 2024). As the population continues to age, more people will need caregivers to aid with physical or mental health limitations that they may have. As I stated before, the goal should not be to just live longer; the goal should be to live longer and have a high quality of life well into our golden years.

In order to ensure we continue to have a great quality of life as we age, it is important that we take care of ourselves along the way, particularly during the younger years of our lives, so that we can ensure as we get older we are in the best health that we can possibly be in. Here are tips that will help you guard your health and do what is within your power to ensure a better quality of life as you age.

Except for women of childbearing age who may be menstruating, bleeding from any hole in your body is not a good sign and requires immediate attention from the right medical professional. For example, if you are bleeding from a bowel movement, that is not a good sign; if you find blood in your urine, that is not a good sign; if when you brush your teeth, your gums bleed, that is not a good sign; if you're bleeding from your ear, that is not a good sign; and if you're bleeding from your nose, that is not a good sign. All of these things are red flags to you about your health.

The human body was not designed to manage a lot of sugar consumption. If you are consuming a lot of sugar, your body will eventually break down, and when I say break down, I mean you will begin to put on weight, and your body will eventually lose its ability to control the amount of sugar in your bloodstream, leading to other health problems, such as diabetes, heart disease, kidney disease, and other medical issues that we have discussed in previous chapters.

Our creator really did create the ultimate machine in the human body. It is the most remarkable creation in our universe. Like a complex computer or high-tech piece of technology, the human body gives us all types of warning signs when something is not right: swelling or inflammation that will not go away is a warning sign, nausea or vomiting is a warning sign, shortness of breath or fast heartbeat is a warning sign, blurred vision is a warning sign, and blood in your stool is a warning sign. Make sure that you are vigilant about being in tune with your body and what it is saying to you.

One of the most important things you can do for your health is to ensure that you are eating the right foods that will keep your body regular. What that means is you should be eliminating waste from your body every day. If you are not eating the right foods and drinking the right amount of water, your body will not properly get rid of its waste, which can have very harmful and toxic effects on you. If your urine is golden yellow in color, that is a sign that you are not taking in the right amount of fluids, particularly water, which will help to flush out your kidneys and also help to flush your digestive system so that your bowel movements are easier. Your urine should be light yellow in color.

The next time you sit down at the table to eat, ask yourself these questions: are all the foods I am about to consume good medicine for my body, and will they supply any nutritional value for my body? If you cannot answer that question right away with a quick yes, then the foods you are eating are not good medicine and may be harmful to your body and your health.

Clean eating should be your mission for life. You should fall in love and have a relationship with the food labels of the products that you pick up in the grocery store. What I mean by that is you should become intimately familiar with the food labels, the nutritional value, and the serving sizes of the foods that you buy and consume. The fewer ingredients that you find in a product, the closer that product is to its original food source and the better it is for your health. For example, if you pick up a can of tomato sauce in the grocery store, and the first ingredient is not water or tomatoes, then you should ask yourself if this is good medicine. If there are fifteen different ingredients in that can of tomato sauce, then you should ask yourself if this is good medicine. If there are fifteen ingredients in that can of tomato sauce and tomatoes are at the bottom of that ingredient list, put that can back on the shelf and move away swiftly. Good medicine is healthy food, clean and lean food that nourishes our bodies, fuels our metabolism, and moves through our digestive system with ease. It helps us eliminate the toxins that we accumulate from our bodies.

Your heart is a muscle, and like any other muscle, if you do not exercise it, over time, it will not function properly. Physical activity is key to keeping our heart muscle, along with the other muscles in our body, actively lean and functioning at the highest level. Physical activity and sweating are good for the body. When you sweat, your pores open. This is another way that your body eliminates toxins and unwanted waste. Moderate physical activity raises your heart rate and exercises that all-important muscle, the heart. Moderate physical activity will help you to reduce stress and anxiety and support a healthy weight for your body type.

Your mental and spiritual health are just as important as your physical health. You cannot have total health without the mental, physical, and spiritual components of your health being coordinated with each other. If any of these three components of good total health are missing or lacking, it can have a detrimental effect on the other components of total health. Encourage yourself to be optimistic about life and the world around you. If you see the world around you as a full glass of cool, refreshing water, then you will see the world around you at its worst as a half-full glass of cool, refreshing water instead of a half-empty one.

Gratitude and reflection are good for the human spirit and the human soul. You should express gratitude every day that you wake up alive on this planet with the potential to make that day better than the day before. Reflection will help you find ways to be a better version of yourself every second, minute, and hour that goes by in your life journey. You need gratitude, reflection, and determination for the transformational process necessary to send you on your journey to better health and a higher quality of life.

Smoking, alcohol, sugar, and salt (SASS) are human body wreckers. If you have ever met someone who is thirty years old but looks like they are sixty, then somewhere in their life, they have overindulged in at least two if not all the SASS components. If you want to achieve better total health, you must take a minimalist approach to consumption of or indulgence in the four SASS components. A minimalist approach simply means to minimize your exposure to the four SASS components if you indulge at all.

Your journey to better health will require a change in thinking about the way that you approach the food you eat and what its purpose is. The food you eat is for the nourishment of your body and not meant to be consumed in excess. If you overconsume food to comfort yourself during times of stress, depression, or anxiety, then you are destined to consume the foods that make you fatter, sicker, and more depressed. Food is medicine. If you consume the right foods and get the right amount of physical activity, you can appropriately manage your weight, boost your immune system, and avoid the health problems that plague many others in our society.

There are many things in life that we as human beings have no control over. Having said that, one of the few things that you do have control over is what you put in your mouth. That is why I titled this book *Watch Your Mouth*. Your mouth is the main portal of entry to the rest of your body, and the food/medicine that you allow in your main portal of entry will determine your health and the quality of your life over time.

*Remember, you are what you eat,*
*and your food is the first medicine.*

# CHAPTER 11:

# A MESSAGE TO MY YOUNGER SELF

I often think about how great it would be to have the opportunity to go back in time and speak to my younger self. What would I say to him about the up-and-coming me? What nuggets of knowledge and wisdom would I speak upon the younger version of myself? Having spent a little time on this planet, what jewels of information could I provide for my younger self that could potentially alter the course of my life as I know it now? I believe I would speak the type of wisdom and knowledge into the younger me that would have the greatest impact on my physical, mental, and spiritual development. I would talk about how to be more financially literate, how to overcome the fear of failure, how to always try to see the world through optimistic eyes, and how to turn a negative situation into an opportunity for personal growth, development, and better understanding. I chose chapter 11 of this book to be my renegade chapter. I see it as my opportunity to go off script and speak from the perspective of someone who has stood in the arena fighting like a gladiator, doing my small part to create a better world, and become a better person with each passing day. So, I ask you to prepare yourself, as a small portion of this chapter will be about good health and what I would tell my younger self on that topic, but some of this chapter will be about other topics and ideas that I deemed important to relate to my younger self. So, without further delay, let us get this party started.

## HERE ARE THE THINGS THAT I WOULD TELL MY YOUNGER SELF IN NO ORDER

1. Ask yourself, "If you knew you could not fail, what would you do?"

2. There is nothing in the world more important than good health. None of your dreams, goals, plans, desires, or wishes can you achieve without a good measure of good health to take you there.

3. When unexpected events occur, whether good or bad, pause, reflect, and put them in their proper place of importance in your life.

4. Plant your roots deep so that when the storms of life arrive, as they surely will, these storms will not topple you over; you will stand firm like a tree planted by the river's edge with roots embedded deep into solid ground. Your tree may bend, but it will not break or fall to the ground.

5. Go down on your knees every day and show gratitude for the grace, mercy, and favor our creator has poured upon you. Pray for wisdom, strength, courage, determination, and understanding.

6. Be reflective in your daily life and develop the ability to see the world from the astronaut's point of view. When astronauts are in outer space looking back on our planet, they do not see the wars, the disease, the famine, the chaos, and the lack of humanity. What they see is a globe-like figure spinning in the distance with colors of blue, green, brown, white, and gray in a universe of darkness. The astronauts see our planet in its largest frame with no visibility of the calamities that burden us as humans. To my younger self, I say, you must develop the ability to rise above chaos, to understand and get a better perspective on the chaos. The ability to allow your psyche to elevate to that higher level of conscious thought will bring you the clarity you need to develop a way forward and contemplate a more positive future.

7. You must develop the consciousness and ability to put the events of your life into their proper perspective. Only then will you be able to conquer the challenges that this life will bring while keeping a sound mind, spirit, and soul free from the negative forces that surround you.

8. Self-determination is key to your human existence. Self-determination is why human beings on this planet, no matter what nation, race, ethnicity, or culture, are in a constant struggle against dictatorial rule, oppression, and crackdowns on the human spirit and its insatiable longing to live a free existence. If you are lucky, you may be able to count on one or two fingers other human beings on this planet who are willing to lie down and die for you. So, if there are few, if any, people on this planet who are willing to make that sacrifice for you, why would you let anyone decide how you should live your life on the planet? Self-determination is a key part of living a purpose-driven existence while you are here.

9. Be humble, and always radiate optimism. You do not have to apologize for your God-given gifts or any worldly success that may come your way because of those gifts. Just give all honor, glory, and praise to the creator and live out gracefully your life's purpose.

10. Celebrate your uniqueness! No two people are just alike. Even identical twins have unique differences, and that is the way our creator intended it to be. Embrace what makes you different. Develop your consciousness and ability to see humanity in that which makes you different. Your uniqueness and the way you see the world may just one day be a catalyst to change the world for the better.

11. To my younger self, cultivate in your mind the idea that regular physical activity and good, clean eating, as close to the source that Mother Nature supplies as possible, are keys to supporting an excellent quality of life as you continue to age during your life journey on the planet. There is no fad diet, magic pill, facial cream, exercise machine, Botox, compression sock, or any other fabricated item that will help you outrun or defeat Father Time. Father Time is the undisputed champion of our human existence on the planet. Therefore, control what is in your power to control, give your body the physical activity that it needs to function at its peak, and eat clean foods as close to the source as possible. You ask what that means. Simply put, if you are drinking coconut water, then the first ingredient should be coconut and not much more than that. If you pick up a bottle of coconut water and the first, second, third, and tenth ingredients are not coconut, then you are drinking a liquid, but it is not coconut water. Remember, your food is your first medicine, and if you want to keep an excellent quality of life as you age, you must develop good habits

around what you put into your body and how you exercise your body. If you take care of your mind, body, and soul, you will age like an exceptionally fine bottle of wine, not too bitter, not too sweet, but just like our creator intended.

If nothing else, the COVID-19 pandemic revealed how much we as human beings depend on each other for companionship, fellowship, relationship, friendship, and affirmation. We are all in some large or small way dependent on one another to find value, purpose, meaning, accountability, responsibility, and dependability in our lives. So, younger self, in your relationships with others, do your part to put in the work required to keep the relationship thriving and healthy. Be aware that both trust and accountability in a relationship, whether personal or professional, must continually be nurtured by each individual in that relationship in order for it to thrive, and it requires commitment to the journey as well. Lastly, younger self, relationships may potentially require brutal honesty and a willingness to accept and grow from factual critique and to compromise for the greater good of the relationship, that is, if it is worth the effort and time. May the creator continue to pour his grace, mercy, and favor upon you, younger self. Only God knows how much you will need it. I am without a doubt your biggest fan. There is no me without you. Continued blessings.

# CHAPTER 12:

# SAVED ROUNDS

Our creator granted each of us one human vessel in which to live out our existence on the planet. When the human vessel that you inhabit runs its course, that will be the end of your physical existence on our planet. We as human beings have no control over whom we are born to, the environment we are born into, the genetics we inherit from our ancestors and biological parents, or the physical and mental impairments or disabilities that we are born with or may face during our lifetime. There are things in our lives that we can control. One is our outlook and attitude toward life and our existence, and another is the foods that we choose to eat for the nourishment of our bodies. As we each continue to grow as human beings, life will ask us to make choices about who we want to be, how we want to live, what we want to believe, whom we want to associate ourselves with, and what we choose to put into our human bodies.

Processed foods typically include those that come in packaging—a box, a can, or a jar on your grocery shelf or in the grocery freezer, such as frozen pizza. They can also be plant-based products that have added sugar, salt, artificial flavoring, and fats. Meats can also fall into this category if they have antibiotics, hormones, chemical preservatives, and genetically modified organisms (GMOs). A lot of processed meat is high in cholesterol, sodium, and saturated fat. Replacing meat that is processed with other available sources of protein has been, based on research, connected to lower rates of death. Some foods are considered extremely processed if they include preservatives, food coloring, artificial flavoring, and other added ingredients that you have to be a scientist to pronounce. These ingredients are in addition to the artificial sweeteners, high sodium, and saturated or trans fats normally found in highly processed foods. Trans fats, also known as trans-fatty acids (TFAs), are unsaturated fatty acids that can clog arteries, increasing the risk for heart disease—the leading cause of death in adults. Trans fats increase the cholesterol that can clog your arteries, making blood flow from the heart difficult. This raises your blood pressure and increases your risk of stroke. Many of the preservatives mentioned increase the shelf life of the product and improve the taste. Stay away from overly processed foods that have no nutritional value. These foods will affect your body's ability to function the way our creator intended. Processed foods are harmful to your cardiovascular system, your immune system, your digestive system, and all the other human systems that keep your body healthy and functioning properly.

A plant-based lifestyle that is well-balanced can help to reduce your risk of diabetes, hypertension, stroke, premature aging, and obesity. Removing the animal fats and cholesterol from your diet while increasing the fiber, minerals, and nutrients commonly found in a plant-based lifestyle can promote a trend toward better health for you.

Vitamin D is one of the most important nutrients for the human body. Making sure you are getting the right amount of vitamin D can aid your body in fighting off and preventing a considerable number of diseases. Low levels of vitamin D can increase your risk for several forms of cancer common in both women and men, as well as heart disease, osteoporosis, lung disease, multiple sclerosis, and other illnesses. See your primary-care physician to have them evaluate your vitamin D level and make sure your D levels are proper and fall within what is considered the normal range as recommended. Make sure you also get enough calcium. Vitamin D and calcium together supply important nutrients to your bones, skin, nails, hair, teeth, and a host of other bodily functions and organs. Vitamin D is called the sunshine vitamin. Inadequate exposure to sunlight can lead to a vitamin D deficiency, particularly if you are not supplementing your food intake with a vitamin D supplement. You should ask your primary-care physician to order a vitamin D test if you believe your exposure to sunlight is lacking. Vitamin C and zinc are a powerful line of defense for your immune system and respiratory health. Both are powerful antioxidants that can help the body fight off disease.

I really like avocado and eat them often. Avocado is rich in omega-3 fats. You should add them to your food regimen. Omega-3 fatty acids are the good-for-you fats that protect your heart by reducing your risk for cardiovascular disease. You should avoid the omega-6 fatty acids, as they can increase the risk of cardiovascular disease and promote inflammation in the body, which is a precursor for many human ailments. Unlike omega-6 fatty acids, omega-3 fatty acids have anti-inflammatory properties that may help fight disease, boost your mental wellness, and reduce symptoms of inflammatory conditions, such as arthritis. Two suitable places to get your omega-3 fats are olive oil and flaxseed oil. Nuts, such as walnuts, almonds, and cashews, and seeds, such as flax and pumpkin seeds, are also reliable sources of omega-3 fat. I would recommend the unsalted version of any nuts that you consume to avoid increasing your sodium intake. Fresh fish, preferably wild caught and not farm raised, is another reliable source of omega-3 fats. You should do your homework and avoid, if possible, consuming the types of fish that are typically high in mercury.

It is critically important that you keep moving as you continue to age. Regularly getting your body moving makes your heart and arteries age more slowly and keeps the cardiovascular system functioning at peak performance. Physical activity enhances your immune system, protects you from stress and depression, helps you to sleep better, and boosts your brain power. Movement is good for keeping the joints flexible and healthy and preserving range of motion as you age.

A substantial number of adults in the United States have lost some if not all their teeth by the time they reach the age of sixty; a noteworthy proportion of that tooth loss is the result of gum disease and dental cavities. With the ever-increasing amount of sugar consumption in the American diet over the past few decades, it is no surprise that periodontal (gum) disease and dental decay (cavities), the two most prominent diseases of the mouth, that proliferate based on the available supply of sugar that feeds the millions of bacteria in our mouth, have become more endemic.

A heart-healthy diet can also help the environment. Commonly consumed animal products, particularly red meat like beef and pork, have the largest environmental impact in terms of water and land usage. Yes, shifting reliance from meat to plant proteins can help improve individual health and help the environment.

A considerable number of people equate being thin with having good health. Nothing could be further from the truth. The weight loss industry is a billion-dollar industry, and in marketing itself its value comes through the concept of getting you to believe that there's some magical pill or injection for weight loss. The industry is dependent on you believing that there is some magical liquid shake that will help you to miraculously burn the fat away and lose weight to better your health. Your weight management will ultimately be determined by the number of calories you take in, the number of calories you burn through exercise and physical activity of some sort, your mental health and determination to positively change your lifestyle while honestly assessing your love for self, and lastly the types of food that you choose to eat and put into your body. There is no silver bullet to weight loss and weight management. To positively manage your weight, it will require a change in basic assumptions in your thinking and a willingness to make a lifestyle change to affect your health for the better.

In this world of confusion, pessimism, and chaos in which we live our daily lives, it becomes very challenging to maintain a cheerful outlook and sense of optimism. Looking at life from a positive perspective is good for your health. Optimistic people significantly reduce their chance of dying from cardiovascular disease. People who interact with the world through an optimistic lens are more likely to eat a healthier diet and maintain an active lifestyle by incorporating regular physical activity, which can foster a longer life span. Living an optimistic lifestyle does not mean you ignore the everyday stressors that life will bring. Living in the world as an optimist means that you intentionally choose to view the challenges and obstacles as temporary, which will allow you to continue learning and growing with a positive mindset as you journey through the world. True optimists believe they have some level of control over their fate, and no matter what challenges life brings, they will be victorious in the end. I encourage you to practice optimism and protect your health.

One of the hardest things for me to learn was to slow down while eating my food. It required a conscious effort on my part to take smaller bites of food and put down my fork in between bites. What I discovered by eating more slowly was that it gave me the opportunity to enjoy the flavors of my food. I began to eat less and allowed my food to digest properly. Because of this conscious change that I have made, now I feel like I have better control of the foods that I ingest and their impact on my physical health.

I am not a health guru by any means. My methods of preventative medicine and my journey to better health may not work for you. This is my blueprint on my journey toward a healthier me. I am sharing what little knowledge I have acquired with you for the ultimate uplift of our human family. Honestly, my journey to create a healthier me continues daily, and each passing day brings new challenges to overcome. I do use the small victories that I find along the way to continue to propel me forward. If there is something shared in this book that works to help you on your journey to better health, I give praise and glory to our creator. I, like you, I hope, will continue trying my best to find ways to uplift the world around me.

I struggle with my fear of failure, my fear of not being successful in achieving the goals that I have set for myself. Your success, like my success, lies just on the other side of that fear. So let go! Step out on faith, and let's overcome our fears and doubts together. I once heard someone say if your goals and dreams do not scare you, then you are not dreaming big enough.

**The late great Dr. Benjamin E. Mays, the sixth president of my alma mater, Morehouse College, once said this:**

The tragedy in life does not lie in not reaching your goals; the tragedy lies in having no goal to reach. It isn't a calamity to die with dreams unfulfilled, but it is a calamity not to dream. It is not a disaster to be unable to capture your ideals, but it is a disaster to have no ideals to capture. It is not a disgrace not to reach the stars, but it is a disgrace to have no stars to reach for. Not failure, but low aim is sin (B. Mays 2024).

When your fear of missed opportunity and your fear of regret start to outweigh your fear of failure, then you are ready to go, ready for success. I will end this book with a quote from Stuart Chase: "For those who believe no proof is necessary. For those who don't believe no proof is possible" (Chase 2024).

*Remember, you are what you eat,
and your food is the first medicine.*

# ACKNOWLEDGMENTS

I want to personally thank everyone involved in my maturation and evolution over time. I especially thank my parents, John and Betty Prince, and my siblings, Ernest, Sharon, Michael, John, Darryl, and Lynn. Our humble beginnings shaped who we are today. Gratitude to our Blodgett Homes, Harborview, and Hatteras Road family. I am a better man, a better person, a better family man, a better leader, a better husband, a better soul, a better poet, a better writer, a better human being because of the life experiences that I have shared with you and because of your inspiration and influence. I am no scholar; I have no stature or great standing in our world. What I am is a grain of sand, gathered up by the hands of our creator, moistened and molded like clay by the forces shaping my journey and informed by your sentiments, critiques, inspirational words, and actions. For that, I will be eternally humbled and grateful to you all. The wisdom, strength, courage, determination, and understanding that life has provided are gifts from our creator, and my writing would not be possible without the grace, mercy, and favor of the omnipotent architect of our universe. The gift of creativity is uniquely inherent in each of us, but it requires continued nurturing and demands our attention. I give all honor, glory, and praise to our creator for the gift of creativity. I hope that even a single sentence in this book inspires and uplifts you along your life's journey. Time is and will always be the backdrop to the rhythm of life. "Keep moving to the rhythm, and flow with the time." May our creator pour peace, grace, and mercy upon you.

Etavonni, KP

# RECOMMENDED RESOURCES

www.CDC.gov

www.FDA.gov

www.USDA.gov

www.americanheart.org

www.nhlbi.nih.gov

www.nih.gov

www.ADA.org

www.diabetes.org

www.hopkinsmedicine.org/yourhealth

www.health.harvard.edu/staying-healthy

www.eatright.org/nutritiontipsheets

www.Livenaturallymagazine.com

www.nia.nih.gov/Go4Life

www.medlineplus.gov

www.hsph.harvard.edu

www.stroke.org

www.fooducate.com

www.cooksmarts.com

# ABOUT THE AUTHOR

Dr. Kevin Prince is a dentist, public health professional, scholar, writer, poet, strategic thinker, intellectual, and health advocate. His interests lie in the arts, jazz music, chess, fitness, clean eating, and cultural discovery. Dr. Prince is a product of the Duval County, Florida, public school system. He earned his Bachelor of Science degree in biology from Morehouse College (Atlanta). He completed his dental education at the University of Florida, College of Dentistry (Gainesville). Dr. Prince honorably served in the United States Navy, Dental Corps, for several decades and spent extended time in Europe, Asia, the Middle East, the Pacific Rim and here at home in the continental United States during his military service. Coming from very humble beginnings, he believes that the joy of life is nestled in the journey. Dr. Prince views the world with clear eyes, understanding the challenges that we as humans face. He understands that our resilience, human spirit, and creativity are nourished in a place on the other side of fear, pessimism, and doubt. Dr. Prince is an optimist and champion for the betterment of our species and our planet, a candle in the darkness.

# BIBLIOGRAPHY

Agriculture, Food and Nutrition Service U.S. Department of. 2024. *Biden-Harris Administration Announces New School Meal Standards to Strengthen Child Nutrition.* April 28. Accessed April 28, 2024. https://www.fns.usda.gov/news-item/usda-0069.24.

Chase, Stuart S. 2024. *For those Who Believe.* May 27. Accessed May 27, 2024. https://www.goodreads.com/quotes/167757-for-those-who-believe-no-proof-is-necessary-for-those.

Hippocrates. 2024. *Speed.* May 27. Accessed May 27, 2024. https://speed.musph.ac.ug/the-gretaest-medicine-0f-all-is-to-tea...eed-it-towards-achieving-universal-coverage-in-uganda/#.

Ighner, Benard. 1977. *Wikipedia.* February 4. Accessed May 28, 2024. https://en.m.wikipedia.org/wiki/Benard_Ighner.

Institute, Urban. 2024. *The US Population Is Aging.* May 27. Accessed May 27, 2024. urban.org/policy-centers/cross-center-initiatives/program-retirement-policy/projects/data-warehouse/what-future-holds/us-population-aging.

Benjamin. 2024. *It Must Be Borne In the Mind.* May 27. Accessed May 2024, 2024. https://www.goodreads.com/quotes/3235-ti-must-be-borne-in-mind-that-the-tragedy-of.

McMains, Vanessa. 2024. *Gum disease-related bacteria tied to colorectal cancer.* April 2. Accessed April 2, 2024. https://www.nih.gov/news-events/nih-research-matters/gum-disease-related-bacteria-tied-colorectal-cancer.

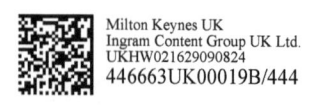

Milton Keynes UK
Ingram Content Group UK Ltd.
UKHW021629090824
446663UK00019B/444